I0419451

Sugar Impact Secrets

Your Journey to Enjoying a Sugar-free Life

By Odelia Rosie

Sugar Impact Secrets

Copyright © 2017

All rights reserved. This book or any portion thereof may not be reproduced or used in any manner whatsoever without the express written permission of the publisher except for the use of brief quotations in a book review.

ISBN: 9781520306872

Warning and Disclaimer

Every effort has been made to make this book as accurate as possible. However, no warranty or fitness is implied. The information provided is on an "as-is" basis. The author and the publisher shall have no liability or responsibility to any person or entity with respect to any loss or damages that arise from the information in this book.

Publisher Contact

Skinny Bottle Publishing

books@skinnybottle.com

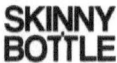

The Bitter Truth About Sugars

SUGAR. Oh, that sweet word! Mouthwatering, pearly white crystals that you and I have both grown to love over the years. Sugar has played a huge part in our modern-day diet --- from your favorite muffins and coffee in the morning to the delicious desserts you indulge in after dinner. And everything in between --- ice creams, shakes, sodas, Butterfingers, Oreo, candies, chocolates --- you name it!

While our early ancestors lived on fruits, fish, and meat, we thrive on sugars. Literally. Almost everything we eat contains sugars, published or sometimes hidden. Food manufacturers use sugar to turn bland tasting ingredients like flour and other processed goods, into "delicacies".

What can go wrong? As long as my meal tastes good, everything is alright!

Really? Well, there's more to sugar than taste. And as you will see in this book, it does you more harm than good.

Sugar is Eight Times More Addictive than Cocaine

I know you've heard about cigarette addiction, drug abuse, and alcoholism. But have you heard about sugar addiction? It's a hard truth but yes, sugar is addictive. Can't believe your eyes? Hmmm...let's talk about addiction really quick here.

The Merriam-Webster Dictionary states that addiction is the *"Persistent need and compulsive use of harmful and habit-forming substances like heroin and alcohol. Upon withdrawal, addicted individuals may exhibit undesirable physiological symptoms."*

Crazy huh? Sugar addiction is on par with heroin and alcohol. And this truth is backed by science! Consider these studies below:

1. According to a study recently published in the American Journal of Clinical Nutrition, food that contains high amounts of sugar can be very addictive. Under the leadership of Dr. David Ludwig, the researchers studied 12 overweight men with ages ranging from 18 to 35 years old. On day one, the researchers gave these men a low sugar milkshake with a glycemic index of only 37 percent. After a couple of hours, they measured the men's blood sugar levels and brain activities particularly in an area known as

the *nucleus accumbens* --- a region in the brain responsible for controlling addiction.

After a few days, the same group of individuals was given exactly the same milkshake in terms of nutrient, calorie and protein content, taste and texture. The only exception was this milkshake contained more sugar than the first (glycemic index equal to 84 percent). The men did not notice the difference. But their brain activities told a different story. The researchers noticed that certain chemical reaction patterns developed in the *nucleus accumbens*. Increased hunger and low blood glucose levels (a physiological response that prepares the body for high sugar intakes) were also evident.

2. The study conducted by Dr. Ludwig and his team isn't alone. In Japan, scientists at the National Institute for Physiological Sciences discovered that consuming food with high amounts of sugar can "trick" the brain and the body into eating more. The research was performed on mice which they found out to release *orexin* --- a chemical that signals the muscles to absorb more blood sugar in the event of a high sugar diet. This is a natural response that keeps the blood sugar levels in the body normal.

So what's wrong? The problems occur when the person chooses to resist the urge of eating more sweets. According to the researchers, the drop of blood sugar levels in the body has two undesirable effects. First, there is an increased craving to consume more sugar. And second, it decreases the person's capacity to resist the urges. In short, it becomes harder and harder to say NO. And like a cigarette addict who needs to smoke or a drug addict who needs to take a hit, the person may need to eat sweets just to feel normal again.

An Average American Eats 22 Teaspoons of Sugar a Day!

Twenty-two teaspoons a day sums up to about 152 pounds of sugar a year. Yikes! And you know what? Significant data suggest that kids eat more sugar than adults. About 34 teaspoons a day, to be precise. If this goes on, 25 percent of all kids in the United States alone may become prediabetic or diabetic teenagers in the next few years!

Unlike overeating, sugar addiction is not emotionally driven. Sugar cravings are caused by hormones in the body. And if left unchecked, it can lead to obesity and complicated health problems like hypertension and diabetes.

Ask Yourself: Am I a Sugar Addict?

It's time to face the bitter truth. *Am I a sugar addict or not?* Fortunately, like other diseases, sugar addiction has its own share of symptoms. Here are some of the most common ones:

- Your body craves for more sweets, especially your favorites when you are bombarded with negative emotions.
- You have sugar cravings and you need to satisfy it in order to experience pleasure and feel normal again.
- The thought of cutting down on certain foods makes you feel sad or at worse, depressed.
- You exhibit no desires to STOP even though your unhealthy eating habits are already affecting your job, relationships, and health.
- You eat certain foods even though you are not hungry.
- Overeating makes your feel exhausted or tired.

If you answered NO to any of these questions, then good for you. But if you answered YES, then we have a lot of work to do my friend. But don't worry. Nothing is ever final. As one of my favorite self-help authors, Brian Tracy puts it:

> *"In life, it doesn't matter where you come from. What's important is where you are going."*

Sugar addiction can be conquered. And in this book, I will show you how.

The 57 Names of Sugar and How to Spot Them

Almost every day, we learn something new about how sugar messes up with our health and waistlines. And you know what's worse? Might food corporations who advertise *"You health and wellness is our primary concern"* come up with new aliases for sugar almost every other day. Check them out below!

1. Agave Nectar

2. Barley Malt

3. Beet Sugar

4. Brown Sugar

5. Buttered Syrup

6. Cane Crystals

7. Cane Juice Crystals

8. Cane Sugar

9. Caramel

10. Carob Syrup

11. Castor Sugar

12. Confectioner's Sugar

13. Corn Sweetener

14. Corn Syrup

15. Corn Syrup Solids

16. Crystalline Fructose

17. Date Sugar

18. Demerara Sugar

19. Dextran

20. Dextrose

21. Diastatic Malt

22. Diastase

23. Ethyl Maltol

24. Evaporated Cane Juice

25. Fructose

26. Fruit Juice

27. Fruit Juice Concentrates

28. Galactose

29. Glucose

30. Glucose Solids

31. Golden Sugar

32. Golden Syrup

33. Granulated Sugar

34. Grape Sugar

35. High-Fructose Corn Syrup

36. Honey

37. Icing Sugar

38. Invert Sugar

39. Lactose

40. Malt Syrup

41. Maltodextrin

42. Maltose

43. Maple Syrup

44. Molasses

45. Muscovado Suga

46. Panocha

47. Raw Sugar

48. Refiner's Syrup

49. Rice Syrup

50. Sorbitol

51. Sorghum Syrup

52. Sucrose

53. Sugar

54. Syrup

55. Treacle

56. Turbinado Sugar

57. Yellow Sugar

You don't have to memorize this list. What's important is you are aware that these sneaky manufacturers are trying to hide as much sugar as possible in your food.

How to Spot Sugars in Food Labels

Fortunately for us, there's a way to spot hidden sugars using the food label. Here's how to do it.

Step 1. Check the "Nutrition Facts" for "Total Sugars"

Nutrition Facts

Serving Size: 6 ounces
Servings Per Container: 1

Amount per serving:

Calories 160	Calories from Fat 25

	% Daily Value
Total Fat 2.5g	4%
Saturated Fat 1.5g	8%
Trans Fat 0g	
Cholesterol 10mg	3%
Sodium 105mg	4%
Total Carbohydrate 26g	9%
Dietary Fiber 0g	
Sugars 25g	
Protein 8g	16%

Vitamin A	0%	**Calcium**	25%
Vitamin C	0%	**Iron**	0%

Step 2. Scrutinize the "Ingredients" List.

The higher sugar is on the list, the more sugar is present in the product

*Percent Daily Values are based on a 2,000 calorie diet. Your Daily Values may be higher or lower depending on your calorie needs.

Ingredients: Dextrose, fructose, honey, invert sugar, raw sugar, malt syrup, rice syrup, sucrose, xylose, molasses, corn sweetener, fruit juice concentrate, high-fructose corn syrup, brown sugar, corn syrup, glucose, lactose, maltose, sucrose, evaporated cane juice, agave nectar, cane crystals, cane sugar, crystal-line fructose, barley malt, beet sugar, caramel.

Step 3. Compare Products

Compare the product with its sugar-free counterpart. For instance, compare strawberry yogurt with plain yogurt. You'll see the difference!

The Fate of Sugar: Understanding How Our Body Uses and Stores Sugar

Our body --- the brain, heart, muscles, liver --- needs energy to do work. And this energy comes from the food we eat. The pizza you ate last night is broken down by your digestive system into its smallest and simplest component called glucose which is, by the way, a type of sugar.

So what happens next?

Glucose is absorbed by the stomach and the small intestine. It is then released into the bloodstream where it can be used immediately for energy or be stored for later.

Insulin, Your Best Friend

The trillions of cells in the body cannot use glucose without insulin. When insulin is released from the pancreas, it "tells" the cells to "open their doors" to let glucose in. Once inside, this simple sugar undergoes complex processes and is eventually converted to energy. Blood sugar level decreases as glucose moves from the bloodstream into the cells.

If you eat a lot of sugary food or a large meal and your body doesn't need as much glucose for its energy requirements, insulin turns the excess sugar into larger packages of glucose called glycogen (primarily stored in the liver and skeletal muscles). Excess glucose is also stored in fat cells called adipocytes.

The burning and storage of glucose are normal processes that occur inside the body. Problems, like the ones you'll read in this book, occur when too much sugar is present or little to no insulin is available (such is the case of diabetes).

Sugars Are Bad? Here are 10 Reasons Why!

Please don't get me wrong. Sugars are good if consumed within one's daily limit. The only downside is that most of us are consciously (or oftentimes unconsciously) taking in a lot of sugar. In fact, studies show that we are consuming an excess of 500 calories a day from sugar alone! And that's very alarming especially if you know what excess sugar does to your body! Below are some examples.

1. Sugar Makes Your Liver Fat

Sugars, fructose, in particular, causes the liver to store more fat. Continuous consumption of high-fructose food may cause fat build up around the liver leading to an illness called nonalcoholic fatty liver disease. That doesn't sound friendly to me!

2. Too Much Sugar May Shorten Your Life

According to recent clinical studies, your likelihood of developing diabetes increases by 1.1 percent for every 150 calories worth of excess sugar in the body! Not to mention other complications like heart disease and cancer. In 2013, another study estimated that over-consumption of sweetened beverages led to more than

180,000 deaths worldwide. In 2010, the United States alone accounted for 25,000 deaths.

3. Sugar Increases Your Risks of Heart Failure

Sugar can increase one's risk for heart disease. Last 2013, a study published in the American Heart Association's Journal showed solid evidence that sugar can mess up with your heart's pumping mechanism. And the culprit? It's a sugar molecule called *glucose metabolite glucose 6-phosphate* (G6P). This villainous compound is responsible for the fatal changes in the muscle proteins of the heart. The study also noted that about half of the people diagnosed with heart failure die in 5 years' time.

4. Sugar Increases Belly Fat

Eewww. Fat! Do you know that over the past 30 years, obesity rates among adolescents have tripled while the obesity rates among children have doubled? There's no need to go to the lab to see what's really happening. A one-time visit to schools, malls or amusement parks is more than enough to see the bitter truth. According to experts, one of the leading causes of fat accumulation in the trunk area of the body is fructose-laden beverages. In 2010, a study in children revealed that excess fructose (not glucose) caused visceral (tummy) fats to mature resulting to a bigger belly and setting the stage for the onset of diabetes, heart disease, and other chronic illnesses.

5. Move Over Hypertension --- Sugar is the True Silent Killer

Yep. Not hypertension but sugar. A silent killer is a disease with no symptoms or warning signs. And in 2008, a study confirmed that sugar fits the role perfectly. Excess fructose (that word again) was linked to an illness known as leptin resistance. Leptin is the chemical messenger that tells you to *"Stop eating because you've had enough!"* For some people, leptin doesn't seem to work while for others, they ignore it. And the result? Overeating which eventually leads to obesity. Take note that we are talking about a silent serial killer here so if you've gained weight without knowing why then you better start checking how much fructose you're taking in.

6. Sugar is Linked to Cancer Production and Affects Cancer Survival

We can't talk about sugar without talking about insulin. Why? Because insulin is sugar's loyal chaperone to the cells. However, when insulin does not work because of too much sugar or other related diseases, the body starts to revolt. One of the many illnesses documented in medical journals is the link between insulin resistance and cancer. Last 2013, scientists discovered that sugars in the intestine catalyze the formation of a hormone called GIP which is controlled by β-catenin --- a protein that's heavily dependent on sugar levels. Researchers found out that β-catenin increases a cell's susceptibility to cancer. Furthermore, high starch and sugar intake decrease the survival rate of colon and breast cancer patients.

7. Sugar Addiction may be Genetic

Do you still remember our little talk about sugar addiction in Chapter 1? According to recent studies, it turns out that sugar addiction may be hardwired at the genetic level. A study of 579 individuals shows that people who consumed more sugar and alcohol had genetic variations in a hormone called *ghrelin*. This chemical messenger is responsible for telling your brain that you are hungry. Malfunction of this hormone results to overeating. It stimulates your brain to "eat more" --- not because you are hungry but because you seek neurological satisfaction (a reward system) through your sweet tooth.

8. Sugar Eats Your Brain

In 2009, a study showed a positive relationship between sugar consumption (particularly glucose) and cell aging. Sugar accelerates aging which could be as simple as a few wrinkles here and there or as scary as a chronic disease. Alarming enough?

Well, there's more to that. Last 2012, researchers found out that the sugar-accelerated aging process affects your brain as well. Increased sugar consumption was linked to memory impairment and the overall decline of cognitive health. In short, sugar eats your brain. And you are not even aware of it! (Well, you are now.)

9. Sugar is Bad for Your Teeth and It Contains ZERO Essential Nutrients

I'm sure your mom told you this the first time she taught you how to brush your teeth but I'll repeat it nonetheless. Bacteria in your mouth celebrate when you eat a lot of sugar. Why? Because it provides them with digestible energy to eat away your teeth!

Furthermore, added sugars such as high fructose corn syrup and sucrose contain ZERO essential nutrients. No vitamins, fats, minerals or proteins --- just 100% energy. No wonder why they are called "empty" calories.

10. Sugar Turns You into a Zombie

What do people say to you every time you need an instant energy boost? *Grab some chocolate bars!* Right? Well, it works but at the end of the day, your body has to suffer the consequences. Sugar-induced energy boosts don't last very long (just around 30 minutes or so). As a result, you will be tempted to grab more and more until it becomes a vicious cycle. Quite ironically, excessive sugar intake also triggers the release of serotonin, a hormone that tells your body "it's time to sleep!"

Our list can go on but I'll stop here. I think they are more than enough to prove that excess sugar is indeed, harmful to the body. So what's next? I bet your other self is now asking: *"How do I prevent sugar from killing my body?"* Chapter 5 has the answer.

13 Practical Tips On How To Reduce Your Sugar Intake

Imagine a life-size statue of yourself made up entirely of sugar cubes and eating it over the next 365 days. That's basically how much sugar you are taking in. No wonder why many people, especially in first world countries, suffer from the harmful effects of sugar that we discussed in Chapter 4.

Although sugar is rich in calories, it has virtually zero nutritional value. Yes, it gives you the energy boost you need but it also:

- makes you fat
- compromises the immune system
- encourages infection and inflammation
- raises insulin levels which stimulates the body to store fat
- promotes asthma, mood swings, hypertension, arthritis and cardiovascular diseases

So before you eat that piece of cake, ask yourself: *"Is it worth it?"*

Saying no to sweets is easier said than done. I understand that cutting out sugar completely is a long shot (who can anyways?). That's why in this chapter, I'd like to teach you 13 easy to follow and practical tips to painlessly and quickly reduce your sugar intake. Read on!

1. Cut Down on Packaged Foods

Spaghetti sauces, salad dressings, pizza crusts and even soups contain sugar. That's why cutting down on processed and packaged products is one of the best ways to reduce your sugar intake. As much as possible, cook at home. If you are making your own soup, you'll unlikely be putting a cup sugar in the pot.

2. Throw Away Your Candy Jar

Do you have a candy jar at your living room or on you desk at school or work? Throw it away and I promise, your sugar intake will drastically decrease. If you really want to eat some sweets, indulge on the highest-quality products that you can afford. Why? Because you'll get more satisfaction from one mouthwatering choco truffle than from five awful sandwich cookies. Make it a goal to only eat sweets that you really, really love and don't care about the rest. Obviously, be careful not to spoil yourself as well.

3. Keep in Mind that Free Sweets Aren't Free

Many businesses and offices offer free chocolates, doughnuts, and other sweets to munch on. And human as we are, it is always our tendency to snack on these cheap calories. Before you grab that candy bar at the door, remember that free sweets aren't truly free. At the end of the day, your body will pay the price.

4. Get To Know Your Sugars

Sucrose, lactose, glucose, dextrose, high fructose corn syrup and maltodextrin are all sugars hiding in your food. Increase your awareness by familiarizing the 57 names of sugar in Chapter 2.

5. Stop Drinking Soda

Remember, sodas are one of the top reasons why most people in first world countries are obese. It's so loaded with sugar and empty calories that experts dubbed it as liquid candy. Don't consume soda as a beverage. Instead, think of it as a special treat that you only drink on special occasions. Do you know what's even better? Avoid it.

6. Be Wary of Your Breakfast

A sugar-loaded breakfast will unbalance your system and offset your energy for the entire day. So better stay away from doughnuts, cakes and milkshakes like frappuccinos and smoothies in the morning.

7. Got a Sweet Tooth? Satisfy it Naturally

Natural sugars are not super healthy but they are better than fructose, dextrose or other empty calories. When you are craving for something sweet, indulge on fruits, maple syrup, molasses, and fruits. These natural sweeteners don't only contain a burst of flavor but also beneficial vitamins that you can take advantage of.

8. Caffeine? Go Black!

Can't miss your coffee? Resolve to drink your tea and coffee without milk and sugar. Go pure black and never go back! Doing this will save you a few teaspoons of sugar each day and money. It's definitely cheaper (and cooler) to order a black coffee than a grande cappuccino with caramel, chocolate drizzle, and whip.

9. Eat Gum But Choose the Natural or Organic Ones

I have a habit of eating something sweet at the end of each meal. If you are like me, you'll find it better to keep a handful of your favorite natural or organic gum for dessert. This will satisfy your sweet tooth and the "chewing" will keep your mouth occupied for a while. If you're used to conventional gum, check out your local food store for healthier options.

10. Eat Regularly

Don't miss a meal. Studies show that not eating regularly causes a drop in blood sugar levels making you feel hungry and increasing your cravings for sweet snacks. Of course, don't forget to include whole foods like fruits and veggies in your diet. These ingredients contain less sugar than processed ones and pose no metabolic issues for a normal body. And oh, natural spices like cinnamon, cloves, cardamom, coriander and nutmeg naturally sweeten your meal without the unnecessary calories. Don't forget to use them in preparing your food!

11. Take Vitamin and Mineral Supplements

Nutrient deficiencies increase cravings. If you want to cut out on your sugar intake, make sure to take good quality multivitamin supplements. They don't only improve your overall health, nutrients like chromium, magnesium and vitamin B3 also improve your body's ability to manage and control blood sugar levels.

12. Move Your Body

I can't stress enough the importance of exercise in maintaining good health. Moving your body --- dancing, doing yoga or other physical activities ---- reduces tension and stress. Exercising also gives you an energy boost and decreases your need for a sugar lift. Don't forget to get enough sleep as well!

13. Distract Yourself

Usually, cravings last for 10 to 20 minutes. When it "attacks", distract yourself by doing something else. For instance, go for a walk or take a shower. Eventually, the cravings will pass. The more you do this, the easier it becomes to manage your cravings.

8 Reasons Why I Love Being Sugar-free!

My first few weeks of cutting out on sugar almost drove me crazy. At one point, I even relapsed and bought a frappe at Starbucks! Luckily, I was able to convince myself to keep going. My curiosity to find out how a reduced sugar intake will improve my health and overall well-being and foster increased satisfaction and happiness won. Today, I'm reaping the benefits of my sheer determination. And if I only have three words to describe my experience, I would say "I love it!"

Below are 8 reasons why I love being sugar-free!

1. Save a Lot of Money

Reducing your sugar intake is not only good for your body, it's good for your budget too! Before, I always find myself spending any spare change I have on my favorite sweets --- banana cake (which pairs perfectly with my morning tea), doughnuts (during my office break) and macaroons (for dessert).

Being sugar-free kept me from buying impulsive sweets. And choosing to cook at home or eat before going out saved me a lot of money! And oh, I now enjoy my new variety of snacks --- fruits, granola or almonds!

2. Blast Those Nasty Fats Away!

Although this is a pretty obvious benefit, weight loss still deserves a space on this list. Since I started cutting out on sugar, I've lost almost 9 pounds already! Yey! Now my old jeans will fit!

3. Better Complexion

Surprisingly, avoiding excessive sugar gave me a clearer skin. Pimples and acne become rare and when I do get them, they're gone in less than 24 hours! Great huh?

4. More Energy

Before, my battery goes red between 3 pm – 5 pm --- forcing me to snack on a chocolate bar to get a quick energy fix. On the other hand, being sugar-free gave me more energy that when I get home from work, I still have the power to catch up with friends or jog with my dog!

5. Increased Motivation to Eat Healthy

The more low-sugar or sugar-free choices I make, the more motivated I am to eat healthily. Why? Because it makes me feel good about myself. I noticed that I become more motivated to experiment with new healthy recipes and to keep pursuing my lifestyle goals. Yes, I know that organic ingredients are sometimes more expensive than processed "crap". But I don't worry. Because the benefits of being healthy are more than what a couple of dollars can buy.

6. Less Snacking and Improved Appetite

Did someone ever tell you that you have the appetite of a pigeon? Since quitting sugar-rich goods, I discovered that my appetite has increased. I now eat seconds and sometimes thirds. You know what's even better? I don't need to snack between meals anymore! And less snacking means less sugary treats!

7. Stronger Willpower

It takes a lot of willpower and determination to become sugar-free. And like the muscles of your arm, willpower becomes stronger every time you use it. Reducing my sugar intake has strengthened my resolve. Instead of relying and caving on my spouse, I am now able to resist temptations almost all the time!

8. Less Anxiety and Improved Mood

Experts confide that sugary foods may cause poor concentration, irritability, anxiety and other emotional outbursts. Honestly, I have anxiety problems too. But since I started cutting out my sugar consumption, I become less anxious and more satisfied with life despite the curved balls that it occasionally throws at me. Issues that constantly worry me in the past gradually disappeared. And yes, I am HAPPY.

Other Benefits!

Obviously, there's more to being sugar-free than the 8 reasons I listed above. Here's a trick, go back to Chapter 4 and imagine not going to experience all the reasons why sugars are bad!

Making low-sugar food choices and restocking your pantry can be pretty overwhelming at first (trust me, I've been there). But don't let these seemingly insurmountable challenge overcome you. As you continue to make correct diet choices, you will eventually find yourself getting more and more comfortable with this new shopping and cooking routine. No effort is wasted. It's all worth it!

Stay Away! 12 Sugar-rich Food to Remember and Avoid!

Do you know that the World Health Organization recommends that children and adults cut their sugar consumption to not more than 10% of their total calorie intake?

For women, the American Heart Association recommends that women consume less than 25 grams of sugar a day (6 teaspoons) while for men, no more than 38 grams (9 teaspoons). How many teaspoons of sugar do you put in your morning coffee? Truth is, you might be eating more sugar than you realize. And if you are not careful, you are setting yourself up for complicated health problems in the future. To help you, here are 12 sugar bombs to remember and AVOID!

1. Yogurt with Fruit

"Wait! Yogurt is supposed to be healthy right?" Yep. But not the ones with added fruits because they contain tons and tons of sugar. Want a number? Up to a staggering 19 grams per cup! If you really want to indulge on yogurt, buy a plain variety and add your own sliced fruit. And oh, don't forget a drop of honey to sweeten it up --- naturally!

2. Canned Soup

Canned soups are notorious for their high sodium content. But do you know that they're hiding whopping amounts of sugar in that can as well? For most canned soups, sugar acts as a preservative to extend the product's shelf life. Depending on the brand, you can find up to 15 grams of sugar per cup! So when shopping, check the labels or even better, make your own soup at home.

3. Salad Dressings

Salads --- kale, spinach, lettuce, all the green stuff --- are healthy until you squeezed that bottle of salad dressing. Depending on the brand, you can find up to 4 grams of sugar for every tablespoon of dressing, especially on fat-free or light varieties. Manufacturers use sugar to make up for the flavor lost by reducing fat. The best choice? Enjoy your salad with a squeeze of fresh lemon juice and a dash of olive oil.

4. Tomato Sauce

Many of us buy tomato sauces in jars from the supermarket because they are more convenient. But would you trade convenience to health? Tomatoes have an acidic taste so manufacturers often use sugars to enhance flavor. Also, like in salad dressings, sugar acts as a preservative that keeps jarred sauces fresh. Most brands sneaked up to 24 grams of sugar per cup of tomato sauce!

5. Bread

Some brands contain up to 2 grams of sugar per slice. And yes, that includes some whole wheat varieties. Don't get me wrong though, you can still enjoy your sandwiches --- just make sure to use bread with no whole wheat flour and little to zero sugar in the ingredients.

6. Granola Bars

Granola bars are either healthy or glorified candy bars. If you are not paying close attention, you might end up getting hooked on disguised-as-healthy granola bars with up to 9 grams of sugar per bar! The ingredients? My best guesses are corn syrup and enriched white flour. If granola bars are your favorite (like me), snack on bars that have no more than 35 percent calories from sugar. Or better, snack on whole nuts and fruits!

7. Dried Fruit

Okay, I just wrote fruits up there. When I say snack on fruits, I mean fresh fruits. Dried fruits sound healthy but actually, they are not. For example, a handful of dried cranberries can pack up to 29 grams of added sugar! Can't resist it? Play it safe by looking for all-natural alternatives --- that means only the fruit is in the ingredient list; no added sugars whatsoever. It might be quite challenging to find an all-natural variety so your best option is still to snack on whole, fresh fruits.

8. Orange Juice

All-natural orange juice? Seriously? Unfortunately, yes. Although this breakfast favorite doesn't contain any added sugars, it still packs up to 9 grams of sugar per glass. That's almost as much as a glass of soda! Instead of drinking orange juice, the United States Department of Agriculture (USDA) recommends eating the whole orange for the extra benefits of dietary fiber. The same recommendation applies to other whole fruits like grapes and apples!

9. White Flour

Do you know that white flour has the same effect on your blood sugar level as refined sugar? During flour processing, the good substances like bran and germ are removed from the final product. Manufacturers then add vitamins to it and sold it as "enriched" to the unsuspecting public. Crazy huh? So be wary especially because white flour is one of the key ingredients of most bread, pasta, pies, pancakes and cake.

10. Carbonated Drinks or Soda

Do I have to write more? A can of soda holds up to 15 teaspoons of sugar and almost 150 empty calories. Not to mention caffeine and loads of artificial preservatives, flavorings, and food colors. Even diet sodas are not exempted --- manufacturers simply replaced sugar with dangerous sweeteners like aspartame! *How could they? Oh, for the name of Profit!*

11. French Fries

French fries are simply deep-fried starches --- sugars. A single serving may contain up to 200 calories from sugar and almost no nutrients. Studies show that one French fry is as bad as one cigarette! Remember that!

12. Ice Cream

Oh no, not my favorite ice cream! Almost every ingredients used to make ice cream --- dry milk solids, high fructose corn syrup, and hydrogenated oils --- are bad for the body. I love how an anonymous author described ice cream: *"It's [ice cream] is just a concoction of unhealthy chemicals presented in an appealing packaging designed to entice the unsuspecting public to their death.*" One ice cream bar contains as much as 17 teaspoons of sugar.

The list ends here but not your quest for sugar-free food. As a rule of the thumb, make it a habit to scrutinize food labels and watch out for sugars. Remember, the higher sugar is on the list, the more sugar is present in the product! Before you proceed to the next chapter, I think it's high time to go back to Chapter 2 and familiarize yourself with sugar and it's 57 aliases.

6 Healthy Sugar Alternatives

Since sugar and artificial sweeteners are bad, does that mean I have to live a rich, good, healthy life deprived of anything sweet?

No! Of course not! You're a human being not a cat (do you know they can't taste sweet? They don't have the taste buds for it. Poor thing!). Anyways, back to topic.

There are a lot of natural and perfectly healthy sweeteners out there. As a matter of fact, I'm compiling you a list right now. So read on get acquainted with these 6 healthy sugar alternatives!

1. Raw Honey

Raw honey is my favorite! I love it so much that I even eat it by the spoonful! Okay, enough about me. Raw honey isn't just sweet. It's packed with a host of wonderful health benefits. It's steaming with antioxidants, boosts the immune system, promotes better digestive health and is a natural antibacterial. More importantly, raw honey is known to balance blood sugar levels and stabilize blood pressure!

2. Stevia

Stevia is probably one of the most famous natural sweeteners in the world. Its sweet leaves have been used by humans for hundreds of years --- especially in Asia where it's used as a cure for diabetic patients. Although it has low nutritional value, stevia has zero calories. Do you know what this means? This means that stevia won't affect your blood sugar levels at all!

Commercially available stevia comes in two varieties --- powdered and liquid. I personally recommend the liquid one since it does not contain any other ingredients except for the whole-leaf extract. Powdered stevia, on the other hand, may contain unnecessary fillers.

3. Date Sugar

In a nutshell, date sugar is just pulverized dried dates. It's very sweet which comes as no surprise to those who have eaten dates before. However, keep in mind that date sugar does not melt. So you do not want to put it in your coffee or morning tea. Instead, date sugar is great for baking! For starters, just use 2/3 the amount of date sugar in lieu of white or brown sugar in your recipe.

4. Coco Sugar

Coconut sugar does not only have a minimal effect on blood sugar levels, it also contains iron, calcium, potassium, zinc and antioxidants. For those who have not tried it yet, coco sugar tastes like brown sugar. It's not sweet enough for coffee or tea so I often use it in baking especially because it does not mess up with the consistency of the final product.

5. Pure Maple Syrup

This is not the one you used to enjoy with your pancakes --- check the ingredients and you'll most likely see high fructose corn syrup, artificial colors sweeteners, flavors, and colorings.

Pure maple syrup contains nothing but evaporated maple tree sap. And it's not just a natural sweetener. It also contains manganese which is necessary for antioxidant and energy production and zinc which strengthens the immune system.

6. Molasses

Molasses come from sugar cane. It's a thick syrup produced when sugar cane is processed to make brown or refined sugar. Unlike refined sugar, however, molasses is widely known for its significant health benefits. It has been said that 2 tablespoons of molasses hold about 30% of iron RDV for women as well as 14% of copper RDV. Molasses also contain vitamin B6, calcium, and magnesium.

13 Tasty, Sugar-free Recipes

"The healthy man is the thin man. But you don't need to go hungry for it: Remove the flours, starches, and sugars; that's all."

Samael Aun Weor

Apple and Egg Muffins Recipe

What you need:

- 3 tbsps. of warm water
- 9 eggs
- 3 green apples (chopped into half-inch pieces), peeled
- 3 tbsp. of coconut milk
- 2 tsp. of ground cinnamon, divided
- ¼ tsp. of baking soda
- 1 and ½ tsp. of coconut oil
- 1 and ½ tbsp. of coconut flour

What to do:

1. Prepare the oven and preheat it to 350 F. Sauté the 1 and ½ tsp. of cinnamon, coconut oil (or butter oil), water and apples in a skillet until the consistency of an apple pie filling or applesauce (chunky) is achieved. Set aside and cool.

2. Whisk the coconut milk, butter, eggs, and remaining measure of cinnamon, coconut flour, salt and baking soda in a bowl. Pour in the previously prepared apples and mix thoroughly. Please leave approximately ¼ cup of cooked apples for garnishing.

3. Using a spoon, place an appropriate measure of the mixture into muffin tins that have been previously lined with parchment cups. Top each muffin with a teaspoon of the reserved apple mixture.

4. Put the tin into the oven and bake for approximately 40 minutes. Once done, allow to cook for a while then transfer to a cooling rack to finish cooling.

Yields 12 muffins

Healthy Pumpkin Pancakes

What you need:

- Half cup of pumpkin puree (can be boxed, canned or fresh)
- 4 beaten eggs
- A pinch of salt
- ¼ tsp. of baking soda
- 2 tbsp. of butter, melted (you can also use coconut oil)
- 1 tsp. of cinnamon
- 1 tsp. of pumpkin pie spice
- 1 tsp. of pure vanilla extract

What to do:

1. Whisk together the pumpkin puree, eggs, and pure vanilla extract. Once done, sift the remaining dry ingredients (cinnamon, pumpkin pie spice, and baking soda) into the mixture.

2. In a skillet, melt 2 tbsp. of butter using medium heat. Pour the melted butter into the pancake batter once done. Combine thoroughly.

3. Using a spoon, pour the batter into appropriate sizes in a previously greased skillet. Flip the pancakes to the other

side when bubbles start to appear.

4. Perfect when served with sliced bananas and grass-fed butter.

Yields 8 small pancakes

Chicken Egg Muffins Recipe

What you need:

- Black pepper, to taste
- Sea salt, to taste
- ¾ lb. chicken breasts or thighs must be skinless and boneless
- 6 eggs, whisked
- ½ tsp. of garlic powder
- 3 tbsp. of clean-ingredient hot sauce
- 3 tbsp. of butter, melted (you can also use coconut oil)
- 2 tbsp. of green onion, sliced (you can also use scallions)

What to do:

1. Prepare the oven and preheat it to 425 F. Carefully pace the chicken thighs (or breasts) into a baking pan. Sprinkle some garlic, black pepper and sea salt. Put the pan into the oven and bake until the chicken is cooked through (approximately 25 minutes).

2. Once done, shred the baked chicken with two forks. Pour 2 tbsp. of hot sauce and 2 tbsp. of melted butter over the chicken. Make sure that the chicken shreds are evenly

coated. Set aside.

3. Whisk the remaining measure of butter and hot sauce, eggs, black pepper, sea salt and green onion in a small bowl. Pour this mixture into a previously prepared and lined (you can use parchment cups) muffin tins. Fill each cup halfway. Using a spoon, put about 2 oz. of the shredded chicken mixture into each cup. Make sure it's evenly distributed.

4. Put the muffin tin into the oven and bake until the edges of the muffins become golden brown. This would take approximately 30 minutes.

Yields 6 muffins

Tasty Asparagus Soup with Lemon Grass

What you need:

- 1 onion (small)
- 500 ml of vegetable stock
- 1 bunch of asparagus
- 1 peeled clove of garlic, whole
- 1 tbsp. of olive oil
- 1 stalk of lemongrass

What to do:

1. Cut the woody ends of the asparagus, wash and chop into small pieces. Grab the onion and dice it. Leave the garlic as it is.

2. Pour the olive oil into a pan, heat it over medium heat. Toss in the garlic clove, onion and sauté until tender. Add the chopped asparagus then remove the garlic clove. Stir and make sure that asparagus is evenly coated with oil. Sauté for a few minutes.

3. Wash the lemongrass. Peel off the outer layer and bash the stalk to release its flavor (you can use a wooden spoon).

Add to the onion and asparagus.

4. Pour in the vegetable stock into the mixture and heat for around 10 minutes (don't boil) or until the asparagus is firm and tender. Take away the lemongrass and transfer the soup to a blender. Blend until smooth.

5. Add some salt and pepper until desired taste is achieved. Serve and enjoy.

Yields 2 servings

Amazing Fried Egg Crepe

What you need:

- Salt, to taste
- Ground black pepper, to taste
- ½ cup of egg whites
- Fillings (could be roasted asparagus, salsa or guacamole)
- 1 egg

What to do:

1. Prepare a frying pan and spray it with olive oil or coconut oil. Warm for about 30 seconds using medium heat then crack the egg in the middle. Pour in the egg white and spread it evenly across the pan by tilting it in a circular motion.

2. Cover the pan and cook the egg until the egg whites and yolk have settled (approximately 2 to 3 minutes). Cooking time depends on the capacity of your stove.

3. Slide the crepe onto a plate and add the fillings. Season with pepper and salt then roll. Cut into small pieces (if you want) then serve. Enjoy!

Yields 1 egg crepe

Sugar Detox Avocado Toast

What you need:

- 1 tsp. of lime juice
- 4 eggs
- 1 avocado
- Salt, to taste
- Ground black pepper, to taste
- 3 tbsp. of coconut flour
- 1 tbsp. of ghee or more as needed
- Optional toppings (tomatoes, celery, herbs, etc.)

What to do:

1. In a bowl, whisk the eggs and coconut flour until smooth and thick. Add some salt and pepper.

2. Pour the ghee in a skillet and heat using medium heat. Once melted, add approximately ¼ cup of the egg mixture. Cook until golden brown (about 2 to 3 minutes) then flip to finish cooking (about 1 minute). Repeat the same process with the remaining mixture. You can add more ghee as needed.

3. In a small bowl, mash the avocado until desired

consistency is achieved. Pour some lemon juice and season with salt and pepper. Mix well.

4. Spread the avocado mixture over the cooked pancakes. Serve and enjoy!

Yields 4 pancakes

Spaghetti Squash Bolognese

What you need:

- Sea salt, to taste
- Ground black pepper, to taste
- 3 oz. of tomato paste
- 1 spaghetti squash
- Half cup of coconut milk (full-fat)
- 1 finely diced onion
- 1 finely diced celery stalk
- 1 clove of finely diced garlic
- 1 finely diced onion
- 2 tbsp. of grass-fed butter
- ½ lb. of ground pork
- ½ lb. of ground beef
- 4 chopped slices of bacon

What to do:

1. Prepare the oven and preheat it to 375 F. Cut the spaghetti squash lengthwise and remove its seeds and inner portion. Season with black pepper and sea salt to taste.

2. Place both halves of spaghetti squash (face down) on a

previously prepared baking sheet. Put in the oven and roast until the skin starts to soften and squash becomes translucent (about 45 minutes).

3. Cool the squash then scoop out the flesh into a serving bowl. Set aside.

4. Prepare a skillet and melt the butter using medium heat. Sauté the carrots, celery, and onions until tender. Toss in the garlic and cook for another 1 minute. Add the ground pork, beef and bacon to the mixture and cook until browned.

5. Once browned, pour in the tomato paste and coconut milk. Simmer the sauce for 20 to 30 min. over medium heat. Season with black pepper and sea salt to taste.

6. Pour sauce into roasted spaghetti squash and serve. (Note: you can prepare the sauce while the squash is being roasted to save time)

Yields 4 servings

Greek-style Meatballs

What you need:

- Zest of 1 lemon
- 2 tbsp. of extra virgin olive oil
- 2-3 lemons, fresh and thinly sliced
- 1 lb. of ground meat
- ½ tsp. of oregano, dried
- Sea salt, to taste
- Black pepper, to taste
- ¼ tsp. of garlic powder
- 1 clove of minced garlic

What to do:

1. Prepare the oven and preheat it to 400 F. Combine the garlic, sea salt, black pepper, garlic powder, lemon zest, ground meat and oregano in a bowl. Mix thoroughly.

2. Using your hands, form 9 to 12 meatballs (depending on size) and place them on a baking sheet or an oven-safe dish. Top the meatballs with lemon slices.

3. Put in the oven and bake until meatballs are well done or pinkish in the center (approximately 20 to 25 min).

4. Before serving, drizzle the meatballs with extra virgin olive oil. Serve and enjoy.

Yields 9 to 12 meatballs (depending on size)

Spaghetti Sauce for All Noodles

What you need:

- 2 tbsp. of extra virgin olive oil
- 2 tbsp. of coconut oil
- 1 tbsp. of fresh basil, chopped
- ½ cup of diced yellow onion
- ½ tsp. of fresh oregano, chopped
- Sea salt, to taste
- Black pepper, to taste
- 18 oz. of tomatoes, diced
- 2 to 3 cloves of minced garlic

What to do:

1. Prepare a saucepan. Heat the coconut oil over medium heat. Put the onions and cook for around 5 min. or until they appear translucent. Season with black pepper and salt until desired taste is achieved.

2. Stir in the minced garlic and cook for 30 seconds. Put the tomatoes and stir to mix thoroughly. Put some salt and black pepper then simmer for 15 to 20 min. Once done,

toss in the chopped oregano and basil. Cook for an extra 5 minutes.

3. Serve over noodle of choice. For extra flavor, drizzle it with extra virgin olive oil.

Yields 3 to 4 servings

Sweet N' Hot Garlic Chicken

What you need:

- Sea salt and black pepper, to taste
- ¼ cup of coconut aminos
- 1 tbsp. of coconut oil
- 1 finely sliced onion
- 2 pinches of chili flakes
- ½ tsp. of ginger powder
- 2 cloves of minced garlic
- 6 chicken thighs, boneless
- 1 tsp. of white sesame seeds

What to do:

1. Prepare oven and preheat to 425 F. Melt the coconut oil in a pan. Place the chicken thighs and season with black pepper and sea salt. Cook the chicken until the skin becomes brown (around 5 to 6 minutes). Set aside.

2. In a small bowl, combine the garlic, sesame seeds, coconut aminos, chili flakes, onion, sea salt, black pepper, and ginger.

3. Flip the chicken (skin side up) then drizzle with sauce

mixture. Make sure the chicken is evenly coated. Put the pan into the oven and bake until internal temperature is 165 F. (approximately 30 minutes).

4. Serve and enjoy!

Yields 3 servings

Broiled Salmon with a Dash of Lemon

What you need:

- 1 lb. of wild salmon
- 1 tsp. of rosemary and salt blend
- 2 tbsp. of butter (you can also use coconut oil)
- 1 lemon

What to do:

1. Prepare the oven and preheat to a low broil setting.

2. Grease the baking dish with butter or coconut oil. Put the salmon slices and sprinkle with rosemary and salt. Coat the top of salmons with extra butter or coconut oil then top with lemon slices.

3. Put the dish into the oven and broil until salmon is cooked (depending on your preference). This would take around 10 to 15 minutes. Thicker slices may take longer time than thin slices of salmon.

Yields 3 servings

Note: For the rosemary and salt blend, follow the directions below:

What you need:

- ¼ cup of coarse sea salt
- ½ cup of dried rosemary, ground

What to do:

1. Run all ingredients through a food processor. Store in a Ziploc bag or in a jar for future use.

Dill Vegetables with a Dash of Garlic

What you need:

- 4 to 6 carrots, cut into long thin strips
- ½ tsp. of garlic powder
- Sea salt and ground black pepper, to taste
- 1 tbsp. of garlic ghee
- ½ tsp. of dried dill
- 1 cup of zucchini, cut into long thin strips

What to do:

1. Melt the garlic ghee in a skillet using medium heat. Place the carrots and sprinkle with ground black pepper and sea salt to taste. Cook the carrots until edges start to brown and until the color becomes brighter (around 10 minutes).

2. Together with the garlic powder and dill, add the zucchini into the pan. Combine thoroughly and cook for additional 3 to 5 min or until the edges of zucchini start to brown.

3. Once done, transfer the veggies to a plate and serve.

Yields 3 servings

Red Cabbage, Onions and Apples Combo

What you need:

- 1 tbsp. of coconut oil
- 1 green apple, sliced into very thin pieces (matchstick-sized)
- ½ head of thinly sliced red cabbage
- 1 thinly sliced onion
- 2 to 4 tbsp. of apple cider vinegar, unfiltered
- 1 tbsp. of rosemary salt blend (refer to broiled salmon with a dash of lemon recipe)

What to do:

1. Put the oil in a pot. Sauté the onion until the color becomes translucent. Toss in the cabbage and cook until soft.

2. Sprinkle with rosemary salt blend and pour in the apple cider vinegar. Continue cooking until everything is tender.

3. Add the apple slices and cook until fork-tender. If mixture appears too dry, just add more apple cider vinegar.

4. Serve and enjoy!

Yields 4 servings

Win a free

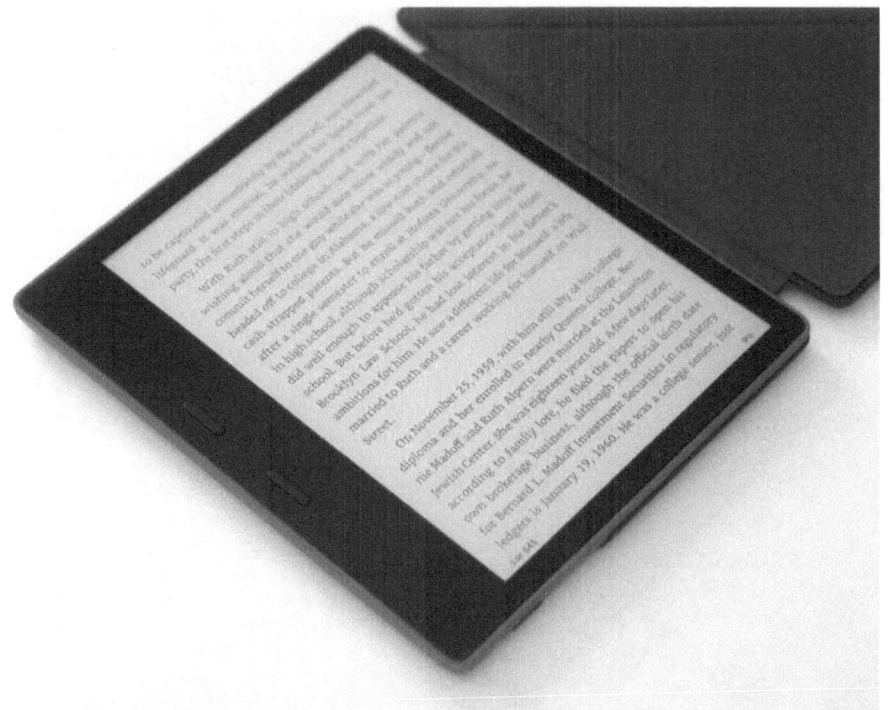

kindle
OASIS

Let us know what you thought of this book to enter the
sweepstake at:

http://booksfor.review/sugarimpact

www.ingramcontent.com/pod-product-compliance
Lightning Source LLC
Chambersburg PA
CBHW030522290526
45786CB00004B/1584